A Lifetime of Healing

Also by Crosslin Fields Smith

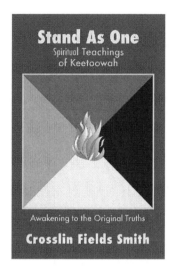

Stand As One
Spiritual Teachings of Keetoowah
Awakening to the Original Truths

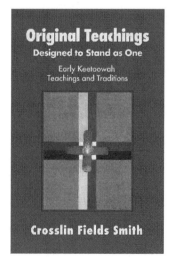

Original Teachings
Designed to Stand as One
Early Keetoowah Teachings and Traditions

Both books available through Amazon.com,
your local library, or your local independent bookstore.

A Lifetime of Healing

by

Crosslin Fields Smith

Dog Soldier Press
P.O. Box 1782
Ranchos de Taos
New Mexico 87557

Library of Congress Control Number: 2023902335

Printing: Ingram Sparks and Kindle Direct Publishing

Print ISBN: 979-8-9874524-4-8

ePub ISBN: 979-8-9874524-5-5

Kindle ISBN: 979-8-9874524-7-9

Editor: Clint Carroll, Ph.D.
                   Associate Professor
                   Department of Ethnic Studies
                   University of Colorado, Boulder

Transcriber: Dr. Jody E. Noe, M.S., N.D.
                   Natural Family Health & Integrative Medicine, LLC

Front Cover Photo Credit: Crosslin Fields Smith, Eagle Release Ceremony
                                Photographer unknown

Book Design and Layout: Ananda M. Sundari
                                AlchemyArts
                                AlchemyArtsllc.com

A Lifetime of Healing

In Memoriam,

Glenna Elizabeth (Foster) Smith

(September 19, 1929 - October 11, 2022)

To my beloved wife, friend, partner, mother of our children,
grandmother, and great-grandmother of our clan.

Love forever,
Crosslin F. Smith

The title of this book was gifted by Pat Gwin.

Table of Contents

A Lifetime of Healing

In his third published work, Crosslin Smith, Elder and Spiritual Leader of the Cherokee Nation, gives us a fascinating collection of short stories drawn from his lifetime of healing in the traditional Keetoowah way. These stories and reflections help illustrate Keetoowah Cherokee teachings of unity and connection - to each other as human beings, to the Creator, and to the land and all life. Combining personal accounts, memoir, guest testimony, and a transcribed interview, this book of healing stories is presented for all to read and reflect on the meaning of Keetoowah Cherokee Original Laws and the universal spiritual source that Crosslin draws upon in his practice of traditional Cherokee medicine.

Clint Carroll, Ph.D.
Associate Professor
Department of Ethnic Studies
University of Colorado, Boulder

Foreword

"First, do no harm." That is the promise embodied in western medicine's Hippocratic Oath. In the oft-misunderstood world of Cherokee Medicine, stories of conjuring and hexing seem to be as prevalent as stories of healing. Fortunately, spending a few minutes of time with one of our most revered Cherokee healers, Crosslin Fields Smith, will immediately dispel such misconceptions. It will also teach us that long before the concept of western medicine ever existed, Cherokee Healers operated under a code of never doing or wishing harm. That ill will would only inflict harm on the source. Cherokee Medicine and its practitioners, like Crosslin, focus solely on healing.

As Principal Chief of the Cherokee Nation, I have invited Crosslin to provide his blessing for many of our new facilities. Upon each occasion, he continually emphasizes the tenets of Cherokee health and healing. The theme of altruism is one that pervades every presentation given by Crosslin. For a lifetime of healing practice, his cultural wisdom, and his commitment to serving the Cherokee people, Crosslin was bestowed the distinction of Spiritual Leader of the Cherokee Nation.

In the early days of the Indian Health Service (IHS) establishing a presence at Cherokee Nation, it struggled to establish trust with the very citizens it was charged with serving. A young Crosslin, already well versed in Cherokee Medicine, was able to bridge the gap between two worlds that were seemingly at-odds. Not only did he have the trust of the traditional Cherokees but he quickly gained the respect of IHS medical staff.

Soon, Crosslin was granted an office within an IHS health facility. With his presence, Cherokees, historically wary of outsiders and unaccustomed to western medicine practices, were first greeted and treated by a person they both new and trusted.

Along with providing healing practices that were accepted by the Cherokee citizens, Crosslin was also able to educate them about the western methods that could lead to a healthier life. Many IHS patients were treated in methodologies of both medicinal systems. While the IHS providers often lamented that Crosslin was getting better results, he always encouraged the patients to utilize and embrace both systems. The early efforts by Crosslin helped lay the foundation of the exceptional health care system Cherokee Nation has today.

Crosslin is and will always be a healer and spiritual leader. His practice has expanded in many ways: he welcomes all people who seek his help, and he has become known for his participation in academic research, leadership programs, and other educational endeavors.

The Cherokee people are eternally indebted to Crosslin for his lifetime of selflessly sharing his gifts and knowledge. He has recounted many of his healing stories within this book, and it is the work of a true Cherokee National Treasure. I hope you enjoy reading this book as much as I did.

Wado, Crosslin.
Chuck Hoskin Jr.,
Cherokee Nation Principal Chief

Prologue

The stories in this book relate some of the experiences I have had during my lifetime as a traditional healer. Some might call them miraculous. It's true that I have helped people in critical condition to get well, whether that be mentally, physically, or spiritually. And I was born with certain gifts that have put me on this path of healing and that I use in my work. But I present these stories to show you what can be accomplished when we adhere to the ancient Keetoowah mindset and teachings - to stand as one with all people and obtain a perfect state of mind in all that we do. We maintain and keep our heritage by practicing a perfect state of mind. Through this practice, we are kind and considerate to all Creation. That's the model that you want to follow. This model personality represents the Original Laws. You don't have to be at a ceremonial ground or at church to do that. We take this practice with us wherever we go. Things happen for your benefit when you're that way.

In this way, we might say that the stories in this book are not about miracles. They are examples of the Creator's ability to help us, which has always been there. It is through this unbroken connection that we must strive to uphold the Original Laws, which I have written about in my previous books, *Stand as One: Spiritual Teachings of Keetoowah* and *Original Teachings: Designed to Stand as One*. This book of healing stories is meant to accompany the other two books and to help explain the spiritual knowledge contained in them.

A Lifetime of Healing

"The Source of Spiritual Power"

According to my father, Stoke Smith Sr., when he lectured the congregation at the ceremonial grounds, he would relate to the ancient times, when the Creator lived amongst our people and all people. At that time, he would say our ancestors were immortal, which means they were like God. In this era, our people lived in a perfect world. You might say it was like the Garden of Eden. They didn't need for anything. They were strong, healthy, and intelligent. They were aware of the whole universe. Later, the people became mortal and started misusing the teachings. This story relates to all races of peoples. The early teaching given to all people by the Creator comes from the perfect world. In our method of healing, we truly become one with the Spirit of God. We stand as one with all Creation. It is the Creator that does the healing; we are only workers following the early teachings.

In my young days, I witnessed my father perform many healing procedures. This is how I acquired my skills for healing. Dad told me that when you perform these healing methods, you relinquish everything that's in your personality. No emotions, no ego, nothing on your mind except what God gave you when you were created: God gives love and his Spirit to all that comes into this world. This is the state of mind the healer is required to maintain. You become a conduit, and God does the healing.

Back about forty years ago, I got a call from Sandra Fox, who was employed in Washington DC. She related the problem that her daughter Trina, about 10 years old, had a serious bladder problem. They had been to several professional medical people, to no avail. In the process of our conversation over the telephone, I was doing a spiritual diagnosis over

Trina's ailment. I received a very strong positive answer that I could use the Spirit of God to heal her affliction. Taken from this spiritual diagnosis, I told her mother Sandra that she needed to come to my home along with her daughter. My diagnosis indicated that I could help her. They came and they were required to stay with me for four days. In those four days, we did spiritual healing methods by water and herbs. Within four days she'd become healed. Not too long ago, I received a letter from Sandra who is now living in Albuquerque, New Mexico. She sent me a picture of Trina and said that she was still doing well, and that the healing was a success. Below is a copy of her letter sent to me in August of 2021.

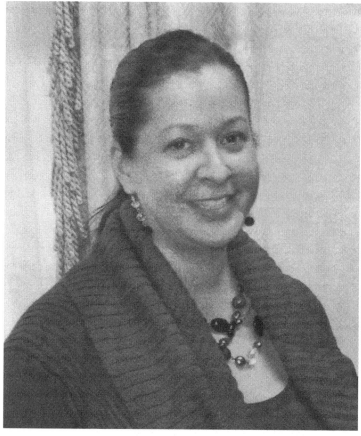

Trina (Fox) Locke, photo courtesy of the Fox family

In 1986, Trina L. Fox (now Locke) was almost ten years old and was living with her parents, Drs. Dennis and Sandra Fox, in Annandale, Virginia. They lived there because they worked in Washington, DC. Her father was the assistant Director for BIA education, and her mother worked for ORBIS Associates, a Native-owned contractor that provided technical assistance and training to and for American Indian Title IV (Indian Education Act) projects in the eastern United States.

Trina is a member of the Mandan, Hidatsa, and Arikara Nation, and is a descendent of members of the Oglala Lakota Nation. She had just started the fifth grade. She was a healthy young girl; however, she was having bladder infections that wouldn't stop. Her parents took her to a pediatrician who prescribed antibiotics that would seem to arrest the infection, only to have it returned shortly thereafter. This cycle recurred and recurred.

Trina's mother was introduced through her work colleagues to Mac Hall, Cherokee, who provided training and programs to foster wellness, physical and mental, for Native youth. Mac recommended that Trina be treated by Crosslin Smith, Cherokee healer.

In October, Trina's mother took her to see Crosslin at his home in Oklahoma. Trina remembers staying at Crosslin and his wife's house for a week; medicine; prayer ceremonies, especially at dawn; Crosslin taking her horseback riding; she thinks she had her 10th birthday celebrated there, on or near Halloween - the same day as Crosslin daughter's birthday; a wonderful pheasant dinner.

Trina's treatment was successful. She had no more bladder infections, even to this day. The Foxes have stayed in touch with Crosslin's family over the years as lifelong friends. They have called upon Crosslin to help them with other needs - physical and spiritual - and are so grateful to him.

"I Found from the Earth…"

The story of Dwayne Wolf, a male Cherokee tribal member about 40 years old, had gone to Claremore Oklahoma Indian Hospital because he had an infection on his right foot. The whole foot had turned black, evidently with gangrene from his diabetes. The diagnosis from the doctor at the Indian hospital proved out to be gangrene infection so therefore the doctor recommended amputation for his leg to be taken off just below the knee. He refused the surgery. It is unknown how he found out about my work, but he came to my house and my spiritual reading and diagnosis gave me a strong indication that I could help him. I found from the earth, a certain plant that would subdue the gangrene. A tea was made from that plant for him to take a cupful in the morning and evening. Before he consumed the first gallon, he was told to come back and get a second prescription. At that time there was an indication of the discoloration disappearing from his foot with lines of clearing. When he consumed the second gallon, all the discoloration had gone. In addition, the doctor had told him he had a weak heartbeat, and when he went back to see the doctor about the amputation, the doctor was overwhelmed. He saw there was no infection, and his heartbeat was strong.

The doctor wanted to know what Dwayne had done to get well. Because of the confidential nature of our practice, he did not want to relate what kind of medicine he had been taking. He finally gave in to the doctor's interest and told the doctor he took Indian medicine. That just increased the doctor's interest in wanting to know what was in the medicine. It becomes a very difficult communication problem. It seems that the medical doctors don't understand the Spirit that comes from the perfect world. In other words, a spiritual approach to diagnosis is lacking in the medical field.

"I May Know Someone Who Needs Your Help"

There was a time when a certain person worked in the care of children. Most of them had been referred to an institution by the court. And the person in charge would have to care for the children. The caregiver was a Native American spiritual person. During the night, when the children had complaints—maybe they had headaches, or stomach aches, or were just lonesome, the caregiver would perform healing methods for the children, and it would work. The children, whenever their guardians visited them or they went there, would relate the healing methods their caregiver would do for them. When the guardians visited, they came looking for the caregiver. They even went to the head of the institution looking for that guy.

The head of the institution would take a negative attitude because the parents were looking for the caretaker. He even stated, "I don't know why they are looking for him when I'm the head of the institution." There came a meeting called to explain to the head the healing methods the caregiver used on the children. And the head of the institution asked, "How does one contact you for this help? The Indian parents are saying they don't understand." The caregiver said to the head, "well, we have telephones, we have letters, we have oral communication for that."

Later on, the head of the institution related information to the caregiver of the children, saying, "I may know someone who might need your help." In a spiritual manner, the caretaker knew that the head was referring to himself. So, again he came to the caretaker saying, "I am the one who needs your help. I have a very serious problem and I've come to think that my spouse is having an affair with another man. I plan to kill them both, and then kill myself." According to his readings and diagnosis, the response of the caregiver to the problem was that the head of the institution needed four spiritual treatments. It is very likely that these treatments were the original baptism from the perfect world, or what we call the Holy Water Treatment. He received the four treatments. Later on, the caregiver got a letter from the head of that institution, signed as Reverend. Those treatments helped the man become a Christian minister.

"You Must Have Love and Care for All Mankind in Your Mind"

Several years ago, a man who was on probation from larceny of various things. This character was a rough individual who would rather strike with his fist to settle any kind of difficulty. He was brought before me and in my communication with him I addressed him according to his character: "You never listened to the good instruction given to you. This one time, you better listen. If you don't, you are heading for ten years in the penitentiary." While on probation, he drove into the trailer lot and hooked up to a trailer and drove away with it. This is why he had to go to court. It turns out the trailer he took was on consignment and it was owned by a police officer. I told him, "boy, you better straighten up. When you took this medicine, you must have love and care for all mankind in your mind. You need to go to an anger management and rehab to straighten up your mind and when you go to court tell the judge you did that." He presented his case to the judge and the judge told him, "Go back to that rehab before I change my mind." He was released. That's just an example of some of the problems that come to me in my work.

"Maybe the Creator Would Help Him"

Another case was brought to me several years ago. A half Cherokee, half Hawaiian man had been charged with first degree murder. He was a member of the Hawaiian gang in Los Angeles. They got into a conflict with a Black gang, and there was a gang fight. One boy was killed from the Black gang. I recommended that he take the cleansing treatments so that maybe the Creator would help him. He was charged because he was a gang leader, but no one knew who afflicted the death blow to the person who died. For that, he was put on probation and still comes to see me. That was over twenty-five years ago.

A Lifetime of Healing

"It Was You…"

A truck driver somewhere down near Del Rio, Texas stopped at a truck stop, took a shower, and thought he'd have a cool drink—a beer. He walked to the bar, and there was a man sitting there. The man looked at the truck driver, and told him, "You need some help." The truck driver bought the man a beer, but he never did touch it. After a while, the truck driver looked back to the man at the bar, and he was gone. The truck driver, being part Cherokee, called Cherokee Nation and told them a little bit about what happened—that he supposed he needed some spiritual help.

Someone at Cherokee Nation referred him to me. He drove his truck to my house, and when he walked in, he stepped back. His eyes got big. I said, "What's the matter? Come in, sit down." He said, "It was you that was in that bar." I have been told several times that I have appeared to people like that in hospitals and other places. And again, it may not be me that's doing it. The Creator could be using another character who's more qualified, so to speak.

"To Stay on the Good Road"

As a Cherokee spiritual worker, I have come across many afflicted people. One gentleman I remember well. An ex-Marine, a Vietnam veteran, came to me for help with post-traumatic stress disorder. Others he had seen suggested it was the effect of agent orange. In the process of diagnosing his affliction, it was apparent that the strongest symptom was emanating from a negative energy cast against him by a Vietnamese medicine man. My readings from crystal divination showed this medicine man sitting cross legged on the floor of a seven-level temple. He was smoking a pipe with a long handle. In that manner, he was casting, possibly, a justifiable action against all veterans: a spell that brings sickness to the enemy. I say justifiable, because in their own mind, they base their action on the fact that horrible things happened to their people. And yet, our practice, in its true way, does not retaliate. We do not entertain such satanic ways, as you might call them.

The treatment we call the Holy Water Treatment is designed for individuals like this veteran to stay on the Good Road—the White Road. In this manner, I sought to remove from his body all the negative energy cast upon him by the medicine man. I gave him four treatments to free him from whatever it was that was seemingly making him live like a Vietnamese. After the second visit, the veteran broke down. He said to me, "I have never told anyone what happened in Vietnam."

He related to me what had happened. After coming across a straw hut, his company formed a three-man team to investigate the potential threat.

As the middle man, he had the job of kicking in the front door to the hut. The other two in the company were to make sure the sides of the hut were free and clear. When he kicked in the door, a woman and three kids with their hands up were lined up next to the wall.

Not long before that day, the man had witnessed a member of his party killed by an enemy sniper who had hidden in a fox hole covered with straw. Out of the corner of his eye, he saw the straw move, and without delay, he opened fire and accidentally killed a baby. The woman attacked him, and he again opened fire and killed them all. This is the terrible thing he had bottled up in his mind.

After receiving spiritual counseling, he broke down shaking and crying. He had finally told someone what had happened. He could now begin his path of healing from this traumatic experience.

"I Was Here to Help
the Cherokee People"

In the early 1960s, I was employed by the Bureau of Indian Affairs. I was the Boys Advisor at a small Indian boarding school in Greasewood, Arizona. W.W. Keeler, chairman of the Board of Phillips Petroleum, was the presidential appointee as the Cherokee Chief. He asked a BIA employee out of Muskogee, Oklahoma to come and interview me for possible employment with the Cherokee Nation. Jack Allison, who represented the BIA of the Cherokee Nation, interviewed me. The interview went well, and I was asked to come home to work for Cherokee Nation. Mainly, what they liked was that I was bilingual and well educated academically, as well as in the Cherokee culture. I was employed as a resource officer for the Cherokee Nation. It became my job to inform the communities in the fourteen-county area of the Cherokee Nation. At that time, the Cherokee Nation needed someone to explain how the $14.4 million was to be used that the tribe had won against the U.S. government. We held many community meetings. Out of those meetings resulted the first form of elections within the Cherokee Nation since Oklahoma statehood in 1907. In these meetings, community representatives were elected. These representatives would be responsible for attending all Cherokee Nation executive meetings. It became their job to collect information from the Cherokee Nation and go back to the community that had elected them and give the information back to that community.

W.W. Keeler gave voting rights to the representatives on all issues concerning the Nation. I was very popular with the community, which caused some difficulties. Some officials, like the General Counsel, became fearful of my popularity, thinking I had ulterior motives to become Chief. This was not true - I had no interest in being an official of the Cherokee Nation. But it was hard for some to understand that I was here to help the Cherokee people to the best of my abilities. Because of that problem I inherited, and because of the big business of Cherokee Nation, there was only two of us - Ralph Keen as the business manager and I as the resource officer. That was a major problem. When we asked for more employees for the business of the Cherokee Nation, we could not get help. It became clear to me I needed to get out. For that reason, I returned to a law prep school at the University of New Mexico. That was my way out.

A short time after that, certain people went to the state penitentiary. They went to prison for larceny of the Cherokee properties. I passed the law entrance test and was accepted by the University of Tulsa Law School. My calling was not to be an attorney, confined to four walls. I actually did that to get out of what was happening in Cherokee Nation. My calling was in the Spiritual Realm. In that calling, I supported the chiefs by performing Spiritual rituals such as the water blessing, our holy water baptism.

In that manner, I supported Chief Ross Swimmer. He was a very important Cherokee Chief and was a key helper to my brother, William Smith, when William was involved in a federal criminal investigation. My brother also practiced traditional medicine. He was helping a man who had been wrongly accused. Because he succeeded in helping the man evade capture, my brother had become targeted by the FBI. Federal agents were preparing a warrant to arrest him for harboring and abetting a fugitive. We had to move fast to bring him to court for a preliminary hearing before the warrant was finalized. William was working in Arkansas at that time, and Chief Ross Swimmer took his private plane to bring him back to Oklahoma. We got him to the hearing in time and the charges were dropped. To this day, I still appreciate and honor Chief Swimmer as one of the best Chiefs the Cherokees have ever had. He had faith in our traditional people, who could see the truth and were trying to help an innocent person.

I also assisted Chief Wilma Mankiller, as well as Chief Bill John Baker. In my view, Chief Baker accomplished more than all the other chiefs for the Cherokee people. He was truly a good chief and he also models our Keetoowah teachings of treating all people with kindness and respect. Chief Baker gave me many honorary awards, including the Cherokee National Medal of Patriotism, but the one that was the greatest is the title of Spiritual Leader of the Cherokee Nation, which I hold today. From the current Chief, Chuck Hoskin, Jr., comes the highest honor given to me by my people, the Cherokee National Treasure Award. In his statement from 2020 he said, "there will never be another person like him."

One of my clients was visiting my home, in my medicine room, and saw a large picture of me. He looked at my door where the Universal Mother, Father, and Child Gods are imbedded. He looked at my door and said that I looked like the Male God of my door—the Universal Man. To me, this means that when you become one with all things, you become one with the Spirit of God.

In all that we do, we must carry ourselves this way, lest we fall victim to jealousy, suspicion, and negative competition. The reason for the suspicion

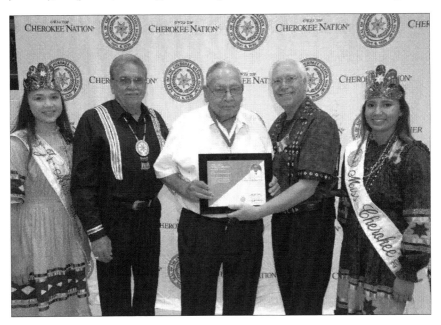

Crosslin Smith receiving the 2017 Cherokee National
Medal of Patriotism Award from Chief Bill John Baker,
photo courtesy of Cherokee Nation Communications Office

from those government officials was that they weren't approaching leadership from a position of selfless service to the people. Having a selfless mindset of service is our traditional way of leadership. We apply this mindset to organize in the best interest of the communities and their needs. When we lose this and get caught up in money and fighting for resources, we lose what it means to be Keetoowah. Some things like money are necessary, but when it sets the agenda, we succumb to the destructive mindsets that damage the people and go against our ways. Top-down leadership can damage the confidence and dedication that individuals may have in our government.

We must never lose sight of our commitment to the Keetoowah mindset that should guide our decisions. If we do, we will have lost our way as a people. We may have success in money and power, but who and what will we represent? This also applies to our interactions with political figures in state and federal government who often don't understand where we're coming from and who try to overturn our rights. In the end, we need to work in partnership. We need to find a way to stand together, not against each other. In this way, we should develop a model from our cultural and spiritual patterns. If people would adopt this, we wouldn't have the problems we have today.

"You Have to Walk Hand in Hand with Your Fellow Man"

One time, I was on a field trip with Chief Wilma Mankiller to visit the Bell community. As we drove along the country roads, Wilma started complaining about her irritated eyes. At that point I spotted a sassafras bush. I told her to pull over and I took a green limb about 6-8 inches long and told her to chew the end of that limb and then squeeze that saliva into her eyes. That gave her instant relief. Many healing methods I offered and performed for many people in the Cherokee Nation. At the beginning, it was very difficult for people to conceive our ancient spiritual culture, but we have come along way with our people accepting our ancient spiritual culture.

We have come to learn certain things that are written in the Christian Bible: for example, somewhere around Psalms 23: 4, it states, "Yea though I walk in the valley of the shadow of death I will fear no evil for thou art with me, the rod and the staff is our comfort." Before that was written in this bible, our ancestors actually performed that through the sacred wampum belt. On that belt, there are two stick figures of people holding hands. This means that you have to walk hand in hand with your fellow man. And try to stay on the path, the white strip that connects the earth and heavens. All spiritual practices are to walk together with one another on the Good Road. If you are on the Good Road, you fear no evil, for God is with you. This information from the wampum belt and the bible are the same thing, which means our ancient people performed what was written in the bible before they ever knew of that book. This means the Ancient Ones represented what the Christian people were trying to do.

Not too long ago, I began a dialogue with a Cherokee pastor from Marble City community named Clifton Pettit. Below are his words based on our relationship and spiritual conversations.

Meeting of Two Hearts - Crosslin Smith and Clifton Pettit

Our Creator has brought two men together who share many similarities. In the meetings with Crosslin Smith, Spiritual Leader of the Cherokee Nation, and Clifton Pettit, who Pastors House of Praise Ministries and oversees the Marble City food pantry, it becomes clear that the unity of their message is the building block for friendship.

Unity, the heart of Creator, is expressed by these men who teach the love for mankind outside the race, gender, age, ethnicity, culture, and many other labels we may use. Crosslin Smith's book, Stand as One, has provided the foundation for returning to our ancestral teachings of the Keetoowah, which are in agreement with Creator's words in the Bible, teachings on the Kingdom of God. "When we speak of yesterday, we have in mind all people, all the parts of creation that ever were." This is a strong statement that brings to life the message of unity in the ministry of Clifton Pettit who has taught us to "love people where they are at."

The message of unity has been lost along the way. We are now hearing this message clearly. No matter the color, we must learn to stand as one. This central message can bring healing. This message was given to our people long before the Bible reached the Keetoowah Cherokees.

Crosslin and Clifton share another aspect of Keetoowah teachings, the White Road Wampum Belt.

Long ago, the wampum belts were put away to conform to the European message. Now, they are being returned to our people. As Crosslin explains in his book, the purpose of the wampum belt was to teach our people Creator's message. The White Road wampum belt taught us to extend our hand to those in the dark and help them onto the White Road. Crosslin states, "The only way to be on the White Road is to be one with all creation." The message of the Kingdom of God is noted in the Wampum Belts. These teachings led Clifton to research and have a White Road Wampum Belt designed according to the description. He has used it to bring understanding to many about our purpose together in the Kingdom of God. Crosslin and Clifton are bringing this message forward at this time as Creator is calling us to live in this level of unity where all are welcome to walk this path, the White Road.

The blending of the Ancients' message and the teaching of the Kee-toowah is in line with the Creator's message to many other cultures that have heard from God and understand the working of the Holy Spirit. From Crosslin's book, Stand as One: "The Father, Son, Holy Ghost wampum belt - just know there is a spirit in your body given by the Creator." The teachings of the Kingdom of God, there are many ways the Holy Spirit or Holy Ghost reveals how He assists us, comforts us, and teaches us. Crosslin and Clifton are sharing the same messages that can help us in this present day to live free. In our world right now, you may experience much devastation and pain, but there is a force inside of us that has great power of healing and life called the Holy Spirit.

As we seek the ancient teachings, they will unlock the answers to questions and help us confront the challenges we face with hope and faith. Both the Keetoowah Cherokee and our fellow Christian believers have resources that are placed by Creator for our good and not for harm. Many times, we have forgotten our ways, but Creator is speaking through Crosslin, Clifton, and others to help us reconnect with our ancient messages of unity and spiritual life. The blending of hearts to walk together, sharing the messages of our Creator, is at the heart of this friendship between Crosslin Smith and Clifton Pettit.

We are stronger together walking this White Road.

"Indian Spiritual Health"

During Chief Wilma Mankiller's administration, she gave me the assignment to make myself available for any assistance that the Indian people may need—Indian spiritual health. I was also assigned to visit Claremore Indian Hospital one full day a week, and as well as Hastings Indian Hospital one full day a week. At Claremore, evidently, a good introduction of my work in the hospital was relayed to the director of the hospital. In that respect, all departments within the hospitals were notified that I would be there on certain days. This had not happened at Hastings hospital—they did not know why I was there. In fact, one doctor reported me to the Cherokee Nation for visiting patients in the hospital. It became clear to me that they were unaware as to why I was in their hospital administrating Indian medicine. The executive committee took a positive attitude towards my work. In fact, the doctor that reported me was present at the executive committee meeting, and for the first time the doctor was informed as to why I was in the hospital.

From those experiences I had with Indian clients in the hospital, one example is an elder traditional woman who was hospitalized in Claremore. The dietician came to me and told me the elder Indian patient was not eating the hospital food prepared for her. I took a quick visit with her, and I recognized who she was. She was a very traditional Indian woman whose name was Blackbird. I asked her how she was doing. She said, "They are trying to give me beef for my food."

Traditionally, we don't eat beef. This is an ancient practice by the older Cherokees. By oral stories passed on to me by my father, they respected the cattle to be a chosen animal by the Creator. In fact, it was mentioned to me that the Creator had selected a baby calf to guard his throne. Many of my elders practiced that belief. It would seem like that concept is connected back to the Hindu practice about the belief that the cows are sacred.

I informed the dietician that the reason her patient would not eat was because the food was made from beef. I told her to get some chopped up pork meat, boil it and make a stew with cornmeal. Bring it to that woman and watch what happens. The woman was so happy after eating the bowl of soup, that she smiled and hugged me. This concept of not eating beef is a possible connection for the disease in the cattle and may one day be transformed into the human body. It is common knowledge that the cattle carried a similar disease as COVID-19. In fact, there has been found an inoculation for cattle to keep the disease down, which maybe one of the reasons why our ancient ancestors did not eat beef.

At the same hospital, I visited a Creek Indian patient who was scheduled for surgery for her leg to be amputated because of diabetes. It came to me by spiritual information that she should not go under the knife. I told her as much. She refused the surgery, and that did not go so well with the medical doctors. But in a few days, she walked out of that hospital. This is what is accomplished by spiritual prayer and traditional healing.

"Acts of Healing with Loving Kindness"

On several occasions, I invited a good friend of mine who studied under my teaching and became a Naturopathic Doctor from Bastyr University. I invited her to go on some of these hospital visits with me. From her own accounts following me on these visits, Dr. Jody E. Noe:

As a young apprentice under the instructions of Crosslin Smith, I had the honor of following him on his hospital visits to folks in the Indian Hospitals. Crosslin saw folks for counseling, for prayer, and for healing. On one occasion, we visited an elder man who was at the end of his journey for this physical life. He asked for Crosslin to come and say the last rites for his passing. Crosslin went to the hospital and performed the passing ritual with his eagle feather in hand, standing at the side of the man's bed. You could see the peace on his face as the Cherokee words fell over him and gave him solace. This peace was evident from the prayer, as his anxiety over his transitioning left him and he was able to have a peaceful ending.

On a different occasion, we visited an elder woman in the hospital who had a recent heart issue. I remember Crosslin bringing in a gallon of tea in an old recycled milk jug into the sterile hospital. He brought her medicine we made from the roots that morning. When she saw him walk in with that jug of medicine her face lit up, she said she knew then that she would walk out of that hospital. Crosslin brought the jug in because he knew what she needed before he even went to see her. Spiritual prayer told him what roots to use.

I have seen healings from simple earaches to spiritual cleansings and everything in between—all practiced with the same Spirit of the Creator and the gifts of Loving Kindness brought forward with every healing. Crosslin has traveled not only between the two federally recognized Cherokee Tribes in Oklahoma to do these healings, but with all peoples across all nations. On his 92nd birthday, he was performing healings for a Shawnee council woman. The healing and the performance of those acts of healing with loving kindness has no rest, as Crosslin takes no days off from this spiritual path.

Over the near 40 years we have been together in this work, I have seen many, many of these healings. I attended with my teacher to the Chiefs of the Cherokees through those decades, observing the ancient practices of protection and guidance for the leadership. I have observed my teacher healing the oldest and most infirmed, the poor, those with only what they have on their backs being treated the same as the grandest of Chiefs of Cherokees. All peoples are treated equal and the same in the medicine, in Spirit. Many times, people would call, or come to his remote home in Vian, Oklahoma, looking for healing on all levels. He would ask them to come in and sit down and eat with the family, then would perform healing acts after they were fed and warmed. Using the elements of the Creator, water, heat/fire, wind/air, and laying on of hands, he applied these healing modalities. All based on a donation system of equity.

"If I Had Known This Before…"

A Native Alaskan woman was diagnosed with cancer, and she went through radiation and chemo with no results. They still diagnosed her as having a cancer. They couldn't isolate what part of her body that was afflicted by cancer. And so, it would seem like they had run out of resources. So, they made a referral to the World Cancer Center in Tulsa. It just so happened that one of the students at the Center was studying with me at that time, Dr. Jody Noe. She happened to be the first to review the folder of this woman from Alaska. After scrutinizing the diagnosis and what they had done for her, she couldn't see any more that they could do except to repeat radiation and chemo. So, she called the doctors in and consulted with them. She noted that they would just be repeating the same treatment, so she requested to make a referral to me, and the doctors agreed. They sent the woman down here with a hospital panel. I talked to her and explained what my diagnosis was.

In my diagnosis, I didn't see cancer. But I did see a negative energy that had been applied to her by her own people. Secondly, she had a very powerful spiritual concept within her personality that sullied the chemo and radiation that they gave her, and that's why it didn't show any help. So, what we had to do is to remove those negative factors from her personality and free her from all of this. There were certain things we recommended. I proposed to perform rituals for her to exorcize the negative energy using water and herbal medicines. I said that if she was willing to go through with that, we could perform them that night. Otherwise, she was welcome to return to the hospital. She said she would stay. In fact, she said, "If I had known this before, I would have come here before the Cancer Center." She was a good client, and she did everything I asked her to do. We sent her back to the hospital. In a day or two, I got a call from Dr. Noe. She told me, "I just want you to know none of these doctors can find a sign of cancer in that woman. She's really happy and is on her way back to Alaska." So, what does that story entail? That negative factors afflicted a certain individual. The Western medical doctors don't have any means to handle this. In this case, it's like they were blindfolded.

"There Was Nothing Wrong with Her"

There was a person who was diagnosed with ovarian cancer. When she came to see me, my spiritual reading told me there was nothing wrong with her. I immediately requested for her to have a second opinion, go to another doctor. She followed my instructions. When she went to the second doctor, he gave her a clean bill of health. There was nothing wrong with her. One day I was invited to speak to about thirty or forty doctors from a family medicine organization in Tulsa. I put the question to them, "What's wrong here? Why was there a diagnosis of cancer with the first doctor, and yet the second doctor said there was none?" Unfortunately, someone may have had dollar signs in their eyes. The first diagnosis that recommended chemotherapy, radiation, and even operation, would have led to about $70,000-80,000 in medical bills. My people don't have that kind of money. I'm not against the medical field, but there is something wrong with a diagnosis of that nature.

"He Was Amazed"

Another woman was diagnosed with ovarian cancer. The doctors said it was so far advanced, and nothing could be done. Somehow or another the woman's family found their way to come and see me. My diagnosis confirmed that she did have the cancer, but also discovered that there was a cure for it. I recommended that she take certain herbal teas mixed with a good alcohol, the alcohol only to be a vehicle for that herbal substance to go to all parts of the body, as well as the affected area. I recommended she take four doses. At the end of the third dose, I recommended that she go back to the same doctor and do a re-diagnosis of her situation. She did, and that doctor didn't find any cancer in that woman. He was amazed: "You're clear, you're clean. What in the world did you do?" She said, "I went to a medicine man, and he gave me some tea and told me to take it." And the doctor wanted to know who I was and wanted to know if he could talk to me. "Well, that's up to him," she said. "I don't know if he'll talk to you or not." But she is well. She doesn't have cancer anymore.

"I Had to Be Confident…"

Some years back there was a young girl who was having seizures. During these seizures, she would become several different people through her voice. Her grandmother was part Creek and Cherokee, and she could talk both languages. When the girl was having a spell, she would talk like her grandmother in the Creek language, but, on a normal basis, she didn't know how to speak Creek. Then while she was sleeping, somehow or other, something would use her body. She would be sleeping in one place, but people would see her walking around somewhere else. I guess you would say she was possessed. It took some time before my diagnosis could be confirmed. I had to build a rapport with her so that she felt welcomed, so that she'd feel OK to be with me. She was deathly scared to communicate with a man. That gave me some indication as to what had happened, yet I couldn't tell her. I had to keep facilitating that conversation for her to say things.

By the time the congregation of her church found out that her parents were bringing her to a medicine man, they were totally against it. In a telephone conversation, I could hear them praying against the devil in me. I knew they weren't using their spirit, and I had to be confident that I was using the spirit that the Creator gave me and to stand by that, come hell or high water. We reached a point where she was glad to come to the house, even though her parents had to steal her away from the congregation and come under the cover of darkness.

We got to where we would converse pretty good. I asked her, "When you go into these seizures, do you experience anything?" She said, "Yes, a man appears to me." I said, "Who is he?" She didn't want to say. She knew who it was. She said, "He calls himself Luke." That was my job - to find out who

Luke was. I had a job to do, and we didn't need to go any further. I gave her some protection medication, in the form of tobacco and cedar, for her to use with water. I did my best to find out who this Luke was.

When she came back about the fourth time, I asked her, "Where did you get that name, Luke?" She said it was in the Bible, chapter Luke. She said something happened during a Sunday school class. Somehow or other the Sunday school teacher was absent, so the minister had volunteered. They were studying the Golden Rule of what God had told Aaron and Elizabeth about her having a baby at 95 years old. The teacher was telling the kids that Aaron and Elizabeth did what God told them to do. He said, "When God tells you something, you must do it." So, he used that Golden Rule to manipulate a beautiful twelve-year-old girl. He kept her after class and he told her, you must do what God told me for you to do. He molested her, and there was a split personality created.

For the minister, he feared word that he had manipulated and molested this young girl would leak out, and he recruited his deacons to put that girl down, satanically. They intended to do away with her, to shut her up for life. They were on their way to doing it. That's when I came in and started instructing her on the spirit and giving her four water blessings as an exorcism. The minister died, but I didn't kill him. It was his own doing, and the deacons soon left. That church is still there. The girl is a woman now and has four kids.

In my reflection on this story, it's important to understand that if people come against you when you are using the true spiritual mindset according to the original teachings, they're not necessarily against you - they're going against God's word. And so, the less we think about people doing something negative to us, the better off we're going to be. We just continue the work along the White Road, and in accordance with the true teachings from the Creator.

"A Perfect State of Mind"

In all that we do, in each and every procedure, we try to reach a perfect state of mind. You must not be involved in anything else, except what you must do to heal that person, without interference. When you have that connection, it's not you that heals, it's the one you're connected to that does the job.

Upon finding the method of healing, you must try to find this perfect state of mind. You must know the attitude and the mind of your patient. You must explain to them to try to reach a state of mind of perfection. If we want the healing power to be applied and we must coordinate with the state of mind with the patient. They must be in the same state of mind as you. If you don't, they will take something from you. It is called draining the power. You must eliminate any negative attitude your patient has against you. Some people who want you to help them, really want to take your energy from you. You might know this is the reason why we cross reference and use Psalms 23, verse 4: *"Yea, though I walk through the valley of the shadow of death, I will fear no evil: for thou art with me; thy rod and thy staff they comfort me."*

I was called by the current head of Oklahoma State University health center, for the new College of Osteopathic Medicine at the Cherokee Nation. I was asked to help train the new doctors. I spoke to them remotely by the Zoom app over the computer, at the new facility. They got a lot of instructions from me that are required for people to become good health care providers.

For example, there must be no negativity in our personalities; we should have only loving care in our minds when we do this work. That's how the Creator gives us success in our healing. It's not us, it's the Creator.

One person then told me their sister was in the next building with a bad headache and asked if I could help her. Her name was Kim Teehee, the first

Native American congressional representative to DC for Cherokee Nation. Kim showed up in the parking lot, and I put my hands on her head, no words or nothing. The healing was in my body and my touch was all needed to take away her headache. She's the living proof of what can be done.

To some people, they fail to understand the method of healing that has a powerful purification. Try to have a perfect state of mind for that moment you are practicing these healing methods. For example, some people may be repulsed when they see you spewing water from your mouth into the patients face. If you don't have water, you use saliva. All your fluids, your water and blood, are a spiritual working method of healing. If you succeed in becoming a perfect spiritual model, you don't have to have your patient in before you. They can be anywhere on this earth; the healing can be transferred. Many times, this has happened - healing by telephone, letters, and vision. It's something that is called the Universal Method of Healing. To some people, they have the eyes of the Creator and can have the Vision.

Epilogue:
A Conversation with Students

In November 2021, a group of students from the University of Colorado Law School met with Crosslin at his home during their visit to the Cherokee Nation as part of the implementation meetings for the United Nations Declaration on the Rights of Indigenous Peoples. Accompanied by Professor Kristen Carpenter, the students asked Crosslin about his practice as a medicine person and Spiritual Leader of the Cherokee Nation.

Crosslin Smith: When you run into difficulty or a problem, don't entertain that problem. Let it go. Turn the other cheek and keep moving ahead. That's what my ancestors did. They left Georgia and North Carolina one year before the Trail of Tears. And they were already here when the Trail of Tears took place. The rest of the Cherokees were forced at gunpoint to make that journey. So, that's a little bit of my background. I am a Keetoowah person. The word Keetoowah was given to my ancestors by the Creator. In one of their meditations, when they used to be together as one with all people, they were seeking information and answers from the Creator. In one of those sessions, a low rumbling cloud glowing like a fire came to them, and out of that glowing cloud came the voice of God. It said, "I've heard your prayers, and in answer to your prayer I've placed a sacred plant on the earth for you to use." Here, we have that sacred plant. It is the original tobacco. The Creator said, "when you use this plant, you are to be fully the name I am going to give you. You will be known as Keetoowah."

To be a Keetoowah, you must be a model of creation. You must be a model of the teachings of the Creator. Back in time, when our people were immortal, they were like God in the Garden of Eden. They didn't need for anything. The teachings with this plant and other teachings come from that far back in time. No matter what you do, the Keetoowah concept—you never lose it. It is unfortunate that some of our people who are in charge of the ceremonial grounds are most possessive of that treasured name. They don't like to see their offspring go to academic schools. They say they leave their culture when they do that. But to be Keetoowah, to live by the ancient teachings of the Creator, this, in part, includes love and care. The Creator told the ancestors in the Garden of Eden that each person who comes into this world, his Spirit is a part of them. We should give them love and care. Whenever you use this medicine, you offer it in this way—with love and care for all mankind. You leave no one out just because they went to school, or they did something that wasn't right. The power of that name represents the Creator.

Anytime you have a conflict with another race of people, remember, don't join that conflict. Because those people who are against you are not necessarily against you, they are against the Original Laws of the Creator. If you completely satisfy the spiritual requirements, people who are against you are going against the Creator's wishes. In the end, God's law is going to win out. That is the spiritual justice that is in the makeup of the Keetoowah. The ancestors were told to stand as one with all mankind. All mankind of yesterday, today, and tomorrow. Going back to this sacred plant, the tobacco, in our original prayer, we offer a small amount of tobacco to all the people of yesterday, to all the people of today, and to all the people who have yet to come into the world. We offer it to the earth that the Creator has given us to live on, including all things that live on the earth with us. We offer appreciation back to the Creator. That's the original use of tobacco.

I have done a lot of blessings across the country in the past. The Department of Public Health used to have regional workshops, like in Oklahoma City or Nashville or different places. Every year, they have that workshop. They called me to do that blessing. So, I did a blessing for them with the use of tobacco. And the surgeon general was sitting in the front row, and he was astonished. Because there is a contrast with tobacco products that have a warning sign on it. But, in our tradition, tobacco was never to be smoked—it was made to offer. That is a spiritual meditation. A spiritual prayer. I don't know if you can move up to being a spiritual person. But there are no words in the intersession with God—it's spiritual. Words are interference to the power of the spirit. You have to be a spiritual person to do this. I understand certain things. Very few people come into the world with a gift of this nature.

But I see in the future that we could have the dimension of seven angels in our culture representing the seven clans. The seven medicine people that represent the seven clans must be a model person, each of them. That's what I would like to see happen again at the ceremonial grounds. Hopefully, maybe educated people could represent the clan medicine position. I would even recommend the Cherokee Nation to think about that. To have seven special model people representing the Cherokee Nation. It's very difficult for people to understand. It takes a mighty good explanation for them to listen to you. We hope that even the children will listen to this. The great promise is that even if there are just three good people, they will save the lives of the rest. There's a cross reference to that in the holy Bible. It's called Sodom and Gomorrah. At that time, God still lived with the people. He appeared to the people of that town and was going to destroy them. Someone from the crowd came up and said, "If I find thirty good people, will you spare us?" And God said, "If you find ten good people, I will not destroy you." It is said they could not find even ten good people, so the good God destroyed them. This is the greatest objective, to keep that from happening to this country. This is for everyone because they lost the early teachings from God. The early teachings remind us that it is love, it is the caring for people, leaving no one out.

So, in short, Keetoowah - stand as one. My brother wrote a little bit in a book that I completed. He wrote, "Even if I went to the moon, I would still be Keetoowah." You don't lose those early teachings. If you look on my door, you will see some images. The top one is the woman God. She is almost not mentioned anywhere. In our culture, the Keetoowah culture, that woman is represented by the fire, the Eternal Flame. And to commune with that Woman God, you must be a model person before her. One with all people. You can give her what you want to give her. She is the number one messenger. She will take it to the father. I've heard this many times from elders, the orators who would speak to our people in front of the fire. They always addressed that fire before anything. They come clean. They call it the Red Lady of the Eternal Flame. They were honoring the Woman God through that fire. The one below is the Male God, the one below that is the Child God, which is Christ. That is what it means to be Keetoowah. To be a model person according to the teachings. You can use that anywhere in this world. It's a special gift.

Certain people are born with a gift. Not all people can do what I am telling you to do. But you have to at least try. A special person born into this world is born as the seventh child, one with a veil over the head, and a twin. I was born with all three of these. That gives a person an extra depth of perception, a sight. One who can do a diagnosis just by looking at people. The true things appear in the faces of people.

It took me a long time to find out who I was and what I was. Many miraculous things happened to me. And I still didn't understand how this was happening. For example, a woman from Washington DC who worked in the BIA building, some of you might know that person. Her name is Sandra Fox. She's retired and living in Albuquerque. About forty years ago, after I was well into practice but still didn't understand everything that was happening to me, she told me she had a twelve-year-old daughter that the doctors in the medical field couldn't do anything for. She had uncontrolled bladder problems, and she couldn't go to school; she couldn't go anywhere. It was a bad case for her. During the conversation, I used my pendulum reading and I got a message this way. Then I got a good indication, a good reading. I said, "Sandra you need to come and see me, and bring the little girl with you." They came, and in four days that girl got well.

Not too long ago, she sent another problem. She had another daughter who had a bad gambling problem and she wanted to see if I could help slow her down. At that time, she sent me a picture of that twelve-year-old girl that we doctored. I finally caught on to the power of being a model Keetoowah. It has a built-in healing power if you succeed in honoring all people of yesterday, today, and tomorrow. That power is in that commitment. So, I didn't cure that girl. It was the Keetoowah process, and it was God who did that for me. So, I'm nothing. I just do what I'm supposed to do, and the Creator does the rest. Now, if you are Christian that is what you have to be. But I think people need to understand that we need to practice love for all people. This can eliminate a lot of problems.

In times before, certain things would happen to me. We used to have wood cookstoves, and we burned wood for heat. And we had a team of horses, and a wagon. And we were hauling dead wood to chop it up in the stove wood. We had driven over a rattlesnake. The wagon tongue attached to the wagon. Right below it was this rattlesnake, and my cousin was the first to see it. From the time he hollered, it wasn't me, but I could feel my movement and I reached over the wagon tongue and grabbed the snake by the back of the head and took him back to the bluff where he belongs. Any other time I would just be as jumpy and scared of that snake. Something came into me at that point. The Spirit took over.

Another time, I was at school, at Indian boarding school. I was in the agricultural club. We worked on the farm and went to school half-day. That morning, I worked at the dairy barn milking cows, making cream, separating milk, and I smelled like a dairy barn when I came into the dormitory. It was kind of late. I got dressed in a hurry and got cleaned up. On my way back to school, I had to pass by a fishpond. It was a large fishpond and at night it would glow with different colors from the lightning bugs. There was a flock of birds bathing in that fishpond, and when I got close, they all took off except one. It kept sitting on that lip of the fishpond. I walked up to it. I was carrying books on one side, but it let me pick it up with my other hand, just like that. I'm walking to school and I'm thinking in my mortal way, "Something is wrong with this bird. It must be injured." But when I got to the schoolhouse door I had to let the books go or let the bird go. I wasn't about to throw away my books, so I opened my hand like this, and the bird took off. It flew away—there was nothing wrong with it. That was a turning point for me to understand myself. I'm sitting in the classroom and the teacher is blabbing about something and I'm thinking, how did I do that?

Just when I left the dorm toward the fishpond, I remember feeling good. Light as a feather. I thought, I must've been one with all creation. I was happy. In that state of mind, this happened, and I learned at that point that you have to be that way to do medicine for people. If it's a court case or whatever, it can be done in that state of mind. Many of those types of experiences had to happen to me before I realized who I was. Then I began to be careful that I don't get angry at anybody because it will affect them. You have to be kind and considerate as much as you can. To be the traditional Keetoowah that I belong to. At this point, maybe you have questions? I would like to entertain questions if you have any.

Student: I have a question. What part of the tobacco plant were you showing us? Was that the flowers of the tobacco plant?

Crosslin Smith: They have a lot of seeds on that. You can plant them. See, it's got multiple seeds. It's a very good plant to have around. We still know a lot of medicine from the earth. We even have a plant that will help keep the virus COVID-19 away from you. If you were taking the medicine and you contracted it, you would get through it OK. Many of my people have been drinking that medicine way long before now. There is a history behind it. They tell me that back in 1919, they had a whooping cough epidemic and my uncle said he did spiritual readings. In our spiritual readings, we do a diagnosis whether we have the gift to do the job to find out the source of the problem. To do what we need to help that person. And he said he took a reading. He remembered that his mother, which would be my grandmother Lucy, that she used to collect those plants and make tea. She would give it to use when we had bad colds and stuff. So, he checked to see if that plant would be good against whooping cough. And yes, he got a good reading. He had one of those big salt vat pots. He filled it with water and got a bunch of that plant and put it in there and boiled it and had a gourd dipper. He had the gourd dipper, and the people were lined up that had the whooping cough. They took the medicine, and they got through OK. That's a little bit of history there. That plant, it's called broomweed. It won't work for you unless you were like a true Keetoowah or a true Christian. There's no difference in being a good Christian and a good Keetoowah - they go together like this. There shouldn't be any conflict. Any more questions?

Kristen Carpenter: I have a question. Some of your earlier remarks were about court and how you were working on a court case. These are young lawyers coming up, so I just wonder if you have some more advice for us and what we are doing.

Crosslin Smith: Well, you're still in a growing stage spiritually. You need to be aware of your existence. You might practice being kind and considerate to all people. That is when the Creator can commune with you. Because you have become attached to him. If you realize God gave you the greatest gift of love and care when he brought you into this world, and he also gave love and care to all things on this earth. He gave you a way to realize your connections. For example, you are connected to certain elements whether you like it or not. You are connected to the meanest man in the world with the very air that you are breathing. You can realize and bring yourself to a point connected by the air, even to a belly-crawling snake—he lives by the air, too. If you can be what you're supposed to be, you can handle that. You're also connected to everything by the water—that is why we say the water is sacred. We need to tell the world to quit contaminating our water. That's what's happening, even our enemies would like to poison all the water in this country. We need to realize that, and the thing that will stop it is the loving care even to those people who would harm our water. You are connected by the warmth of your body to all things, the sacred fire—the sunlight. You are connected by the earth, the soil, to all things. They say the original people came from the soil. That our material body will go back to the Mother Earth in time to come. Only the Spirit lives on.

One of the early teachings to all people is that the Creator told them, "I have provided everything for you here on Earth. I have also provided seven heavens after you die." You go to one of those levels, those seven dimensions. People who live by love and care most of the time in their life on this earth get to go to the highest level of heaven. The seventh eternal heaven. People who didn't do so good go to subordinate dimensions, but they are still given a chance. To go on up by the Spirit. The final objective is that seventh heaven. Christians talk about salvation. We Keetoowah have a built-in salvation. Extra mean people go to the bottom heaven. You might say that there is no hell in our culture. We create our own hell.

So, we need to know what we are doing at certain times in our own mind. If you can't comprehend these things, you may not believe what I'm telling you. It may get you in trouble one way or the other. But we hope to remove all injurious concepts in your mind. We do a sacred water treatment, which is the original baptism given to all people in the ancient times.

Letters to the Author

I only met Crosslin once—it was a long time ago at the National Service Learning Conference in Albuquerque. He gave a blessing before the talk I gave, and I am sure, as a result, my talk was inspired! I remember the occasion as though it was yesterday. It was so clear that he was passionate about working, as a Medicine Man, to help his Cherokee people recover from long years of persecution and discrimination. He told me he felt education for the children, especially education about their culture, was really important. And, of course, he cared about the natural world, and understood that only when we become spiritually connected with nature can we be truly whole. Most significantly, he radiated an aura of calm and a deep and spiritual wisdom that made a lasting impression on me. My only regret was that I could not spend longer with him. I wanted to probe his knowledge and get a better understanding of his teaching. But brief though our interaction was, I carry a sense of his love and blessing with me always.

Dr. Jane Goodall, DBE
UN Messenger of Peace
Founder, Jane Goodall Institute

I should open by saying my brother is Mac Hall, founder and head of the National Indian Youth Leadership Program. He has had a long and very important relationship with Crosslin Smith. About ten years ago, I was diagnosed with diverticulosis—it was a severe case and required several surgeries and removal of some of the large intestine and bowel. Needless to say, I was very frightened by this news and didn't feel confident about my survival. I spoke to my brother, and he said he would take it to Crosslin and see if he could help me. I spoke to Crosslin. He has such a calming and confident voice and way of speaking that it didn't take long for me to put my complete trust in his abilities to see me through this ordeal. He told me from the first conversation that everything would be all right and then he would be there with me spiritually through it all. I've never been so comforted and convinced of anything by just speaking with the person. But he is obviously not just a person. He has such power; you can feel it even through the phone. He and I have spoken many times since then and I feel very blessed and honored that he chose to help me, and to show me that things are possible outside of hospitals and doctors and the accepted way of healing.

I will be forever grateful for his healing of my soul along with my body. He is truly a gift to humanity.

Sincerely,

Cynthia Hall-Mohn

Friend and Client

Revered Elder Fields,

I recently read your two books, Stand as One: Spiritual Teachings of Keetoowah, and Original Teachings: Designed to Stand as One, Early Keetoowah Teachings, and write to express my profound gratitude for sharing your sacred knowledge. The two books were gifted to me by Cherokee member and Native American Rights Fund (NARF) attorney Melody McCoy. Your writings on the Keetoowah Original Teachings of the Creator filled me with wonder and joy as did your life story, connection to Spirit, and use of that connection to heal and provide guidance to others. The wisdom you shared through your books spoke to my soul and whispered truths that have long resonated in my heart. Thank you for giving voice to these truths and sharing them with others in service to all people.

Thank you as well for your recognition of my contributions as a NARF attorney in your chapter on "The Importance of Women." Although I recently retired from NARF and the practice of law, I will always be grateful to NARF for providing me with a vehicle to serve Native people. I am content growing older as retirement has given me an opportunity to step into a new way of being in service to my community in ways of Spirit. Accordingly, I humbly seek to fulfill Creator's design by doing the work of surrendering the desires of the ego and awakening to the great mystery. And in doing so, adhere to Creator's Original Teachings as you so beautifully teach.

As an act of reciprocal gifting for the sacred knowledge that you share, I sent you an eagle feather from the Southeast community of Sitka, Alaska. It was dropped on the doorstep of my childhood friend whose grandmother was influential in my awakening of Native identity as an adolescent. I offer it to you in honor of all you have given to those who are suffering and to those who strive to follow Creator's Original Teachings. The smoked dry fish is from this year's catch of King Salmon which was gifted to me by the Native Village of Tyonek; I cured and smoked it this week. The jar of smoked fish was put up last year but continues to hold cycles of life that the salmon people gift to nourish us. The mushroom Chaga was gifted to my daughter for her work as a climate activist; its nectar is good with tea. The other small items are earrings that were made by Native hands and are expressions of our relationship with the natural world.

Thank you again for your wisdom, your kindness, your acts of selflessness, and sharing your lineage. If it would not be too great a burden and if you were taking visitors, I would be honored to come pay my respects in person.

With humble gratitude,

Heather Kendall-Miller
Former Staff Attorney
Native American Rights Fund

Crosslin and I met while working at the Tahlequah Agency, Bureau of Indian Affairs in the Housing Program in the late 1970s. We got to know each other pretty well. I know this by the way he teased me. His humor is in the typical Cherokee style, where words may make fun of a situation but are spoken in good-natured jest.

I grew to have such respect for Crosslin. He is someone I can go to for help whether spiritually, mentally, or physically. He has taught me so much about our old ways. He teaches why Cherokees have been given gifts from our Creator and how those gifts are to be used. He has taught me the Creator is within all of us and how to use what the Creator gave us to help us get through this life. He teaches anyone who will listen how to awaken this gift from the Creator. It isn't easy and only a few can master it.

What I love about Crosslin is his positivity and his willingness to share his knowledge of spirituality and what the Creator gave to us for all who want to learn. He is a truth teacher and always says he is a tool for the Creator. He is one of a kind.

Fan Robinson
Adopted Daughter

I clearly remember waking from the dream that warned me that something was wrong, and that something was probably cancer. I immediately made an appointment to see a physician who, after some tests, a mammogram and biopsy confirmed that I did indeed have breast cancer. I was in a quandary as to what to do, it was a time of great stress, great fear, and great anxiety. I recall the many times that my grandmother would have me take her to the man she called her "Indian doctor" when something was wrong. She knew that the old ways were really the best ways and taught me the same. So I reached out to a friend, Mac Hall, who put me in touch with Crosslin Smith. I called and Crosslin told me to come and visit and that he would do what he could to help me. I actually remembered knowing about Crosslin and how he had helped my close friend Wilma Mankiller with her recovery and knew that he had also helped another man who had cancer. Wilma held him in very high regard.

I was very hopeful. He gave me directions to his home and as I pulled up, there were several people in parked cars who were also waiting to see him, so I took my turn waiting in the car until he came to get me. He was gentle, kind, and straightforward. There was a prayer, we talked, and then he prepared a drink for me and gave me directions on how to use it. He assured me, after prayer, that there would be no additional cancer found. I left him feeling a great sense of relief. I felt that my soul definitely experienced healing and hope the same for my physical body. I drank the drink he prepared and followed his directions diligently. I told my surgeon that I needed two weeks to follow my traditional ways. He was very understanding and said that I should do what strengthened me. Then it was surgery time. I felt a deep inner piece going into that surgery.

After the surgery, my doctor came in with a big smile and said that there was no additional cancer found in the original cancer was gone. In the days that followed, both he and the nursing staff were amazed at how quickly I healed from such an extensive surgery. I was able to go home two days earlier than expected. I will be forever grateful to Crosslin Smith for the spiritual support and healing by the old ways that he provided to me—physically and spiritually. I believe that my life would've been very different, perhaps much shorter, had I not crossed paths with Crosslin Smith. Wado to you, Crosslin.

Pamela Jumper Thurman, PhD
Senior Research Scientist
National Center for Community and Organizational Readiness
Senior Affiliate Faculty, Ethnic Studies Department
Colorado State University

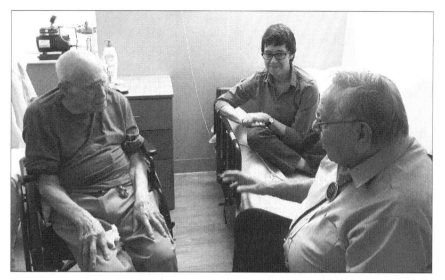

George McCoy, Melody McCoy, and Crosslin Smith
Tulsa, Oklahoma, January 2017

In 1922, George McCoy, Cherokee citizen, was born in Muskogee, Oklahoma to Cherokee citizen parents George McCoy and Sybil Wolfe McCoy. George grew up in Tahlequah and Tulsa. While getting a graduate degree at the University of Tennessee, he met the woman to whom he would be married for life, Sally Richman McCoy, who is a first generation American, born and raised in the Bronx by her parents who emigrated from Poland to avoid persecution as Jews. George and Sally McCoy are my parents. They both were adamant that their children be aware of their heritages.

In 1980, somewhat dissatisfied with his work as a Professor of Psychology at a large midwestern university, George accepted a position with the U.S. Indian Health Service (IHS) as tribes began to contract the operation of their health services under the 1975 Indian Self-Determination and Education Assistance Act. This allowed him to return to Oklahoma, where he could attend reunions at his alma maters Daniel Webster High School in Tulsa and the University of Tulsa. But his favorite reunions were the McCoy Family reunions in Marble City and Vian, Oklahoma. It was through these events that he reconnected with his first cousin, Crosslin Smith, whose mother is Lilah McCoy. They became close, although during George's 25-year tenure with

IHS he rose through the ranks to become the Deputy Director for Behavioral Health, and had to relocate to Rockville, Maryland for a few years. But even after he "retired" he stayed on contract with IHS clinics, again choosing to return to Tulsa, as proof once again that one can take the Indian out of Oklahoma, but one cannot take the Oklahoma out of an Indian.

George was devoted to his work to improve the lives of many, and he is credited with increasing the federal budget for behavioral health services for Indians by 400%. Crosslin similarly is devoted to his medicinal work and spiritual knowledge. I remember my Dad telling me once after a visit to Crosslin and Glenna's that "Crosslin is going to write a book, and I'm going to help him." I thought, what a great pair! My Dad is a good writer (and I mean writer, as my Dad never used a typewriter or keyboard), having written a widely used college text book back in his professor days. Sadly, my Dad's health declined and he moved on to the spirit world before the pairing could happen. So, when Crosslin shared with me recently his frustration that my Dad never got to participate in any of his (Crosslin's) books, and further directed me to write about my Dad for his third book on which he was working, I got the message. Wado (thank you) to Crosslin; George McCoy is delighted and humbled to be with you in this book.

Melody McCoy
Boulder, CO

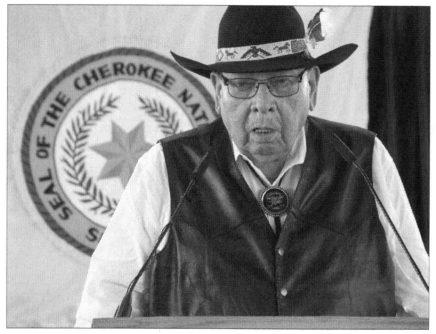

Crosslin Fields Smith,
photo courtesy of Cherokee Nation Communications Office

About the Author

Crosslin Fields Smith was born November 27, 1929, to a traditional Keetoowah family. The members of the Keetoowah Society are best known as the keepers of God's Eternal Flame. Crosslin is a Korean War veteran, having served as a member of the famous 45th infantry, or "Thunderbird" Division of the U.S. Army. He holds a BS in Education and an Elementary & Secondary Teaching Certificate from Northeastern State University and is now retired from a 30-year career of civil service.

Crosslin states that he has always represented the Cherokee Nation. He is the first employee of the Cherokee Nation - from 1964 to the present - as a spiritual resource person. He has worked under Chiefs W.W. Keeler, Ross Swimmer, Wilma Mankiller, Bill John Baker, and the present Chuck Hoskin, Jr. During the reorganization of the Cherokee Nation in the 1960s, Crosslin served as a U.S. liaison officer to his Cherokee people and was responsible for informing them on the status of negotiations between the tribe and the U.S. government. Through the years, he became the tribe's spiritual practitioner, performing blessings at official functions and at the start of new tribal development projects. In 2020, Crosslin was recognized by the Cherokee Nation as a Cherokee National Treasure.

In 2014, Smith was among seven Cherokees honored at the AARP Oklahoma Indian Elder Honors event for their impact on their tribes and communities. A noted keynote and university lecturer, Mr. Smith has standing engagements in the United States and abroad. Crosslin states, "With the highest diplomatic credit and character, I have worked to build a Cherokee Nation for the Cherokee people. I fought in the Korean War. In this war, I represented the U.S. government and the American system. In all of my efforts, I worked to be part of the system instead of against it."

Made in the USA
Columbia, SC
24 March 2023

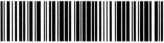

14199613R00039